Brain Wellness - the Book

Migraine Help from a Unicorn Nurse

Practitioner

Mandi Counters, FNP-BC, MSN, RN, SCRN, CNRN
Minneapolis, MN
brainwellnessnp@gmail.com
http://brainwellnesssolutions.com

Mandi Counters © 2023
ISBN: 9798386355173

Acknowledgements

I would be slacking if I didn't give thanks to the people that encouraged me to write this book and believed in me. Huge thanks to Don, Amanda, Eric, Elise, Reyanna, my biological and non-biological children, and all of my colleagues that helped me become the Nurse Practitioner that I am today.

Introduction - Don't skip this!

First off, what is a Unicorn Nurse Practitioner? I have been called a 'unicorn' and adopted the nickname because I realized it fit me pretty well. Let me clarify, I am not a mythical creature with a horn projecting from my forehead, but I do fit the often-second definition of unicorn: something or someone that is highly desirable but difficult to find or obtain. I have had patients and their families tell me that they wish all providers would think like me and actually listen to their patients...hence the hard-to-find desirable something/someone.

So why should this book interest you? For multiple reasons, honestly. Not only have I been a neuroscience nurse practitioner for 10+ years (where I earned the nickname 'unicorn'), but also because I have been a neurology patient for most of my adult life. I began having migraine headaches when I was an early teenager, thanks to my wonderful genetics. I remember when I was growing up, if we went out to eat at certain restaurants (which I will discuss later in this book), my mom would have to pull the car over to the side of the road while we were driving home so that she could vomit because she had developed a migraine. I, like all of my siblings, developed migraines in her footsteps, and my oldest child has so far followed suit. So here's a spoiler - we'll talk about genetics later in this book, as well.

While working as a nurse practitioner in neurosciences, I have had the pleasure of learning from some very experienced providers, both physicians and advanced practice providers (APPs). Some taught me what I didn't want to do in my practice, but most taught me some amazing tricks along the way. I compiled those tricks into my own practice and continued to build on them over the years.

Several years ago, I was introduced to a practice of medicine called 'functional medicine'. Functional medicine looks at the root cause of illness rather than just medicating symptoms. I was so excited when I learned about this branch of medicine because I felt like I was completely born for it. On a daily basis, I help my patients find the "why" behind their neurological disease. I'm not one of those providers who just likes to prescribe medications. Don't get me wrong - there is a place for prescription medications in migraine treatment, but there is an even bigger place for lifestyle management, which is most of what we'll talk about in this book.

So, if you're not interested in making some lasting changes to the way you live on a day-to-day basis and you'd rather just take a pill for what ails you, please put this book back and stop reading, because you won't enjoy this book. On the other hand, if you're open to doing things that come with more positive side effects, please be my guest and read on. This book will be a combination of research and anecdotal information from my experiences as patient and provider. Be prepared to learn things that may contradict what you've been told, as the information in this book comes from my years of experience in medicine, not just from sitting behind a computer making policies for practitioners to follow. That said, thanks for being here.

x

Table of Contents

Chapter 1: What the heck is a migraine?   p.1

Chapter 2: What triggers these awful things?   p.11

Chapter 3: What about genetics?   p.42

Chapter 4: Let's talk about typical medication treatment   p.46

Chapter 5: Now let's talk about non-typical non-medication treatment   p.55

Chapter 6: What foods you *should* eat   p.69

Chapter 7: How about some outside-the-box treatments?   p.76

Chapter 8: What's the risk of not treating?   p.92

Chapter 1: What the heck is a migraine?

Over the years, I have had many people not realize that what they were experiencing was actually migraines. Migraines come in many forms - let's discuss them now, shall we?

The classic symptoms of migraine include throbbing/pounding headache that typically involves one side of the head, with associated sensitivity to light, sound, and/or smell, and causes nausea with or without vomiting. Keep in mind, not every migraine will come with all of these symptoms, as some brains have 'not read the textbook' as I like to say. People may have some, but not all of these symptoms, or may have others instead, which we will discuss momentarily.

Some people have what is called an 'aura', where they have some sort of symptom prior to the headache starting, serving as a warning that the headache is coming. The aura can happen seconds to minutes prior to the headache starting, so for some people, it's not really much of a warning. Not all migraine sufferers experience an aura, and some will have a variety of aura symptoms. It was years into my own journey of experiencing migraines before I realized that I would start yawning prior to my migraines starting, when I didn't even feel tired. Even as a practitioner, I didn't realize this warning sign, so it's not surprising when my patients miss it.

When you Google migraine aura, you will find a variety of reported symptoms. This can include anything from visual changes such as flashing lights, kaleidoscope vision, wavy lines in vision or blurring of vision, to frequent yawning, heightened sense of smell or smelling things that others don't, sudden fatigue, changes in ability to speak clearly, numbness and tingling (which we call paresthesias in medical speak) or even weakness.

Some lucky people have a migraine aura that does not develop into a full-blown headache. On the other hand, some people just have the pain and have none of the above symptoms.

Often patients don't have the classic symptoms of migraine. There are a variety of migraine syndromes that confuse people. We often call these non-typical migraines a very fancy term of either 'atypical migraines' or 'complex migraines'. Real original, right? The atypical migraines often cause people to visit an emergency room thinking something more sinister is happening: a stroke. Two of these major atypical/complex migraine syndromes include hemiplegic migraines and vertiginous/vestibular migraines.

Hemiplegic migraine means: hemi = one half of your body, and plegic = weak. One half of your body goes weak, as you would see if someone was having a stroke. This can range from mild weakness to complete loss of function of one half of your body.

Vertiginous = vertigo = dizziness. The vestibular arteries go up the back of the neck and feed the cerebellum, which is the back part of the brain. That part of the brain is sometimes referred to as the "dizzy center", as this is where our balance center is. So, these migraines can go by many names, including vertiginous migraines, vestibular migraines, dizzy migraines…it all means the same. These migraines make a person dizzy. Patients often use the term 'dizzy' to describe a variety of sensations, but essentially it causes a person to feel off-balance or 'spinny', for lack of better terms. Again, the severity ranges from mild dizziness to severe dizziness where the person can't bear to open their eyes, and can cause nausea, with or without vomiting.

The lucky person that experiences these types of migraines, either hemiplegic or vertiginous, may have these symptoms with or without pain. So that leads to another term used to describe some atypical migraines: acephalgic. Cephalgia is the medical term for head pain, so a-cephalgia is the absence of head pain. These migraines can cause the neurological symptoms just described, but the sufferer does not experience the associated pain. This leads to a lot of emergency room visits for people that believe they are having a stroke. How can we tell it's not a stroke? Head imaging such as magnetic resonance imaging (MRI).

A large population of patients that I have seen over the years describe frequent headaches as feeling like a sinus headache. They have a lot of pain and pressure behind their eyes and around their nose region, so they assume it's sinus headaches. After years of working with patients, however, it became clear that most of these people were actually experiencing migraines, as they may have some of the associated features described earlier in this chapter, but people didn't recognize the features.

Migraines often last hours but can last up to a few days at a time. Regardless of the length of time, the migraine is considered one 'episode'. When you see your provider, they often ask how many migraines you have in a month, but we also ask how many headache-days you experience a month. So, some patients may experience 1 migraine but 3 headache-days, because the migraine lasts for 3 days. That's just as miserable, if not sometimes more miserable, than someone who has 3 migraines that combined create 3 headache-days.

Migraines are more likely to occur in females but can also affect males. There is a hormonal component to migraines, so a good percentage of women experience 'menstrual migraines' or migraines that occur at certain times in their menstrual cycle. This could be either during ovulation or during the actual period portion of the menstrual cycle. Women can also experience a change in the characteristics of their migraine as they progress through menopause. Sometimes migraines decrease or go away altogether, but other times they worsen in frequency or intensity, or even take on a different form completely. A woman who has experienced typical migraines all her life can suddenly start having complex migraines.

Someone who experiences migraines for the first time should have a complete evaluation to identify (as best as medicine can) the cause of these wonderful new experiences. This generally includes head imaging (preferably MRI as we can get more details of the brain with an MRI than a CT scan), and ideally blood testing for vitamin levels. A detailed history is incredibly important because history is generally 90% of the evaluation. Generally, by the time I'm done interrogating (just kidding, I'm nicer than that) my patient, I have a good idea of what's going on with them, and any physical exam or diagnostic testing will confirm my suspicions. Occasionally, even the great Unicorn Nurse Practitioner gets stumped, and I run it by one of my colleagues to decide on further testing.

Chapter 2: What triggers these awful things?

So many things can trigger a migraine! One of the first things I always do with my patients is ask them to keep a headache diary. There are multiple trackers on the market these days, both in print form and in apps for your smartphone, where you can track characteristics of your migraines and lifestyle information that may help to identify triggers. Some of the most common triggers that I discuss with my patients are sleep, nutrition, hydration, exercise, stress. So, let's cover each of these a bit more in-depth, shall we?

Sleep. We've all heard that we should get at least 8 hours of sleep at night (in reality, it's more of a range from 7-9 hours), but how many of us actually accomplish this? The statistics are rather grim…only about one-half to two-thirds of adults actually get sufficient sleep. And aside from the hours of sleep we get, approximately one-half of all adults still report feeling tired throughout the day, because we often don't get the right *kind* of sleep. There are different stages of sleep, the most commonly known being REM sleep. REM sleep is important because this is where our memories are formed, and concentration is managed. Have you seen the movie "Inside Out"? I always think of this movie when I think of REM sleep because when the brain shuts down at night, all the colored marbles (in the movie) are shuttled into their respective places in our memory and things are filed for later. If we get poor sleep, this process is inefficient or incomplete and our memory and daily performance will be affected.

We use the term 'sleep hygiene' to describe the importance of healthy habits with sleep, just like dental hygiene when we refer to keeping our teeth clean and healthy. It's another routine that is very important for proper function of our body. Sleep hygiene means that you get regular sleep, you go to sleep and wake up about the same time each day regardless of the day of the week, you are uninterrupted in your sleep, and you sleep in a proper position.

Often, when people don't follow a schedule for sleep, but instead haphazardly go to sleep at various times in the night, or they wake up early during the week for work but sleep in on the weekends, they lack consistent sleep patterns, and the body has a very hard time adjusting to the chaotic schedule. Well, guess what? So does your brain. Your brain likes structure; it likes the ability to perform its usual tasks of filing memories and programming the body for daily activities. When you deprive your body of structure, it struggles to perform adequately. Imagine how you feel when you get a good night's sleep - now imagine how you would feel if you had that every day. Pretty mind blowing if you think about it.

Other considerations with sleep hygiene include sleeping in a dark room - your brain has a hard time shutting down when lights are still on (this sends a message to your brain that it is still daytime). This is why it is so important for night-shift workers to use room-darkening blinds to simulate night-time in their sleeping area. Ideally you go to sleep without the TV on. Even more ideally, you don't watch TV too close to bedtime, or stare at a computer screen or handheld electronic device too close to bedtime. All the blue light we get from these devices messes up our circadian rhythm (the natural sensation in our body of when it is appropriate to be asleep or awake).

A common supplement used for sleep is melatonin - it is a 'supplement' because it is a naturally occurring hormone in our body, with the responsibility of helping us with our circadian rhythm. Again, the blue lights mess up this rhythm, and our brain gets confused on when to release melatonin in the body to help us get to sleep.

The caveat with melatonin is that you can have too much of a good thing. If you take too much, not only can you overdose and develop headaches and fatigue, but it can shut off your body's own production of melatonin so that you *can't* sleep without it. I recommend starting with 1mg in sublingual form (melt under your tongue) as it tends to be more effective at lower doses and works fairly quickly. I do not recommend taking 10 mg regularly, as this is when we get into trouble with 'too much of a good thing', and you definitely shouldn't take more than 10 my daily.

Many people swear by 'white noise' to help them fall asleep. Relaxing music, use of a fan in the bedroom, or calming app sounds/meditations can be very helpful. I recommend setting a timer on them so they will shut themselves off so that the sounds don't accidentally wake you back up later in the night.

My biggest tip for sleep is creating a routine. We do this for children, why can't we do it for ourselves, too? With our kids, we bathe them, we read to them and tuck them in, and we try to do this at the same time each night. Consider any of these things for yourself - take a warm bath or shower before bed, apply lotion, read with a soft light or journal to end your day (adding meditation/journaling to your nighttime routine will help on multiple levels!), drink some calming tea, listen to music or a guided meditation, or any number of other calm, quiet activities that may help you wind down at the end of the day.

What I don't recommend before bed? Don't play video games, don't watch intense movies (I speak from experience, it will lead to very intense dreams that will wake you up), don't stay up past the point where your body says you're tired, and don't drink alcohol right before bed. While people use the excuse that they need a drink before bed to help them fall asleep, the alcohol actually muddles with your circadian rhythm and will make it difficult for you to *stay* asleep. Ideally, you should actually avoid alcohol within 4 hours of bedtime because of this. Water or warm tea is by far a better option (careful not to drink too much so that your bladder wakes you in the night!).

Nutrition. This is a controversial conversation. If you read sources such as dietary recommendations from the WHO and Dietary Guidelines for Americans, you will find a lot of information that contradicts what you read in this book. The information laid out on the next pages are the compilation of years of providing care to patients and educating myself on what is *actually* healthy for us. When I went to nursing school, we were taught things like the ADA recommendations for diet, which at the time followed the food pyramid (mind you, physicians actually get *less* education than nurses when it comes to nutrition). The food pyramid is now a "thing of the past" and we currently follow MyPlate...which still is not perfect. But none of these guidelines actually take individual health into full consideration. There are many theories behind where these recommendations came from, but the least of them, I'll say, is actual worry about individual health.

It has been said that if we all follow the Standard American Diet (abbreviation is SAD), we will all have diabetes at some point, because we eat far too many carbohydrates and sugars in our diet. Most people are familiar with diabetes types 1 and 2, but have you heard of diabetes type 3? Type 3 diabetes is becoming synonymous with

Alzheimer's dementia. There is a clear correlation with too much circulating glucose in the body and development of Alzheimer's. If we can make that kind of connection, it would be a pretty good assumption that decreasing our circulating glucose would be good for more than just dementia prevention, don't you think?

When we talk about nutrition from a migraine standpoint, we need to discuss things that should be avoided as well as things that should be included in our diet. Things to be avoided will vary a bit from person to person, but there are general recommendations we will discuss now, and later in this book we'll talk about what you should include. Remember when I mentioned earlier about keeping a headache diary? One of the things this is beneficial for is identifying migraine triggers in the foods we eat. When keeping a diary, you can either do it retrospectively (think back to what you ate in the last 24 hours or so prior to a headache - this is noted after you experience the headache) or prospectively (keep track of what you eat prior to actually experiencing the headache). Then at some point you need to analyze (review) this data to look for patterns.

    Some common foods that trigger migraines include alcohol (especially red wine), caffeine, aged cheeses, and processed meats (think of a meat and cheese tray, a charcuterie board), foods containing MSG, and artificial sweeteners. Caffeine is a tricky one, however, because many people use caffeine to treat headaches - specifically if you've ever used the over-the-counter medication called 'Excedrine' - it is a combination of acetaminophen (commonly known as Tylenol), aspirin, and caffeine. So, while caffeine is a trigger for some people, it is a treatment for others.

While these are the common triggers, there are also uncommon triggers. One of the most interesting triggers I ever heard from a patient was onions. If that person ate onions, they would develop a headache. I don't recall if it occurred only with raw onions or if that also included cooked onions, but if you've read many food labels lately, you'll realize that onion powder is included in many packaged foods. Some of these food triggers make eating (and grocery shopping) on a daily basis very interesting.

Some of the formerly uncommon triggers that I see more and more commonly include gluten and nightshade vegetables. Gluten has hit a peak in popularity in recent years and has become a bit of a fad diet for some, but this sensitivity is a real thing. While only a small percentage of the population is truly Celiac (has systemic effects from gluten ingestion), there is a growing population of people with non-Celiac gluten sensitivity.

In the United States, we have processed the heck out of our wheat so that it is not the wheat our grandparents, or even our parents, ate. We have sped up the growing process so that we can produce larger quantities of wheat faster, while making it more insect resistant. So, while you're hearing about less pesticides being used *on* plants, there are more being used *in* the plant's DNA in order to prevent loss of crop to those filthy pests.

Gluten generally refers to the glue-like substance that holds food together and is mainly found in wheat, barley, and rye. These ingredients are often found in breads, pasta, and cereal, but can also be found in things you would not expect, such as candies, sauces, and dressings. Another consideration is cross-contamination, meaning how a food is prepared. If you take food that is naturally gluten free and you cook it in a fryer that is shared with non-gluten-free foods, you have now contaminated your naturally gluten free food. So long, simple French fries.

There has been some talk that nearly all people have a threshold for gluten, meaning that at some point in our lives most people will develop some level of gluten sensitivity with our current foods. This threshold can be reached as early as age two all the way up to 99+. Some of this depends on the amount of gluten-laden foods we take in over our lifespan. So, it's quite possible that someone can grow up eating a certain way and still have gluten issues arise later in their life.

    I used to call myself a 'carbivore' because I loved my carbs, and there was no way you were going to take my carbs away from me. Finally, 10 years ago, I decided to just *try* this thing called Paleo diet (a form of whole-food diet where you cut out processed foods and most grains) that a neurologist whom I worked with at the time recommended. He recommended this diet to many of his migraine patients, and they had great success reducing their migraines. Lo and behold, so did I. In a matter of 6 months, not only did I nearly eliminate my migraines, but I also lost 30 pounds without trying very hard (I shed a LOT of inflammation), I had a skin condition that had been present for nearly 20 years that finally cleared up, and I cleared up a lot of brain fog. It would be nearly 8 years before I found out I actually had a Celiac genetic profile.

Nightshade is a family of vegetables (and some fruits...and some spices) that contain a compound called alkaloids. This family includes tomatoes, potatoes (other than sweet potatoes), eggplant, bell peppers (all colors), goji berries, and spices such as paprika and cayenne. Nightshades are considered to be pro-inflammatory, meaning they increase the likelihood that you will have inflammation somewhere in your body. This inflammation generally starts in the gut and spreads elsewhere, which can present itself in many forms including digestive issues, joint pains, and…headaches.

While it's not necessary for everyone to avoid gluten and nightshades, if you are good about keeping a detailed headache diary and can identify these foods as triggering your migraines, it will serve you well to remove them from your diet. So much for those fajitas…

One thing that is clear for any function in the body related to inflammation is reducing processed foods. Processed foods largely includes foods that come pre-packaged, pre-prepared...meaning boxed meals, frozen dinners, and canned foods. In general, this covers everything in the middle of the grocery store. If it comes in a box or jar, it takes some processing for it to be able to sit on the shelf at the grocery store and have any kind of shelf-life (survivability on the grocery store shelf until you come along at some point to purchase it). The chemicals required to keep these foods from decomposing on the shelf are not natural to your body and will do all sorts of interesting things. Some of these interesting things will include triggering headaches.

Hydration. Dehydration (lack of appropriate water intake) is a significant trigger for migraines. Water intake is so important! It's one of those things that is simple, but not easy. Meaning, it's a simple thing to do - add water to your daily intake of fluids - but so many people say they "hate the taste of water" and find it very difficult to add this needed item into their diet. Our body is about 60% water, and so many bodily functions require water in order to work. It helps our joints stay lubricated, it helps our bowels move regularly, and it helps our blood circulate appropriately.

When growing up, we probably all heard the recommendation to drink 8-10 8-ounce glasses of water daily. For many people that is fine, but I've since learned a better calculation for this. You should actually drink about half your body weight (in pounds) in ounces of water. So, if you weigh 200 pounds, you should be drinking 100 ounces of water. Whoa, right? That seems like a lot...and it is. But it's absolutely necessary.

What counts as water? Any clear fluid that does not have caffeine in it (or added sugar). So, that includes plain water, flavored water (as long as it doesn't have a bunch of added sugar or artificial sugars) even if it is carbonated, decaffeinated coffee or herbal teas, or even plain broth counts. Caffeinated teas and coffee don't count because caffeine is dehydrating, so you're defeating the purpose here. Sodas don't count whether they are caffeinated or not, because they have too much sugar (even diet sodas, as they have too many artificial sugars)!

The best thing to do is start with a glass of water first thing when you wake up and keep sipping throughout the day. I generally recommend cutting it off around dinner time (with the exception of taking medications at bedtime if needed) so that you're not up at all hours of the night urinating. Sleep is important, remember?

Don't like the "taste" (or lack thereof) of water? Add slices of cucumber, lemon or lime, or other sliced fruits to the water. You get a hint of the flavor without all the sugar. You can also use essential oils to flavor your water - I like to add a drop or two of lemon essential oil to my water, again for the hint of flavor without the sugar. Looking to 'detox' off some weight after eating too much at a family gathering and get rid of that bloated feeling? Add sliced lemon, ginger, cucumber, and mint leaves to a pitcher of water and let it sit overnight - enjoy it the next day. My oldest son calls this "fancy water" when he comes to my house and finds it in the fridge.

Exercise. This is one topic that people sometimes find counterintuitive because it's difficult to exercise when you have a headache. Which is true. But regular exercise will actually help prevent headaches. Lack of exercise feeds into some of the other triggers we mentioned (including poor sleep and stress), and in general decreases our overall health. Exercise isn't something we practitioners recommend for our own health - it's for yours, too.

There is no right or wrong kind of exercise, there is only the choice of which kind of exercise you like and will stick with. We always hear how regular exercise is good for cardiovascular health -

this is because it's good for vascular health, in general. Migraines involve some degree of vasoconstriction or vasospasm, meaning the blood vessels constrict, or tighten up, and decrease blood flow to a certain extent. Regular exercise helps to keep our blood vessels responsive to changes in pressure and less likely to constrict and affect blood flow.

General recommendations for exercise are to get in at least 30 minutes of exercise most days of the week. Does this 30-minute recommendation have to be completed all at once? No. If you need to do three 10-minute increments during the day, that's better than none. If you're new to exercise, start with walking. You need to walk fast enough to where it is difficult to carry on a conversation while walking to actually get cardiovascular benefit from the exercise. If you're walking a tiny little dog and it has to stop to sniff the entire walk, the dog *may* be getting exercise but you're not. Sorry, just being real.

    The options are nearly limitless on what kind of exercise you can do. Some people insist on going to a physical gym because they need that motivation - at a gym you can find weights, treadmills, bikes, stair climbers, classes like yoga, dance, or other aerobics, and sometimes large gymnasiums where you can play basketball or do rock climbing. Some gyms are more focused on exercise bikes, or heated workouts, or pilates. At the end of the day, you need to find something you enjoy and will continue with.

MANDI COUNTERS, NP

For years, I have done better with at-home workouts, because that has worked better for my family's schedule. There are so many options for this now - you can find free options via YouTube, or you can subscribe to specific companies or apps, where again you can find a multitude of options for workouts. The benefits of these at-home workouts are that you can do them on your schedule, you don't have to travel anywhere, you can't use weather as an excuse not to work out, and if you don't like the online program you're doing, you can switch to another one. If you have physical limitations to working out, you can still find modified workouts that you can do at home, as well.

I, personally, am a runner. I feel like I can solve the world's problems when I'm running. Am I fast? Not anymore. I was when I was a kid, but with my own health issues now, my pace is not award-winning. If I'm feeling stressed, a good run does me wonders. If it's raining out, it's even better, if you ask me. Running in the rain is cathartic.

It's good to get a combination of different exercises, including both cardio (walking or aerobic exercise) and weight training. Weight training is especially important as we age to keep up bone health. Our muscles and bones follow the old adages of 'use it or lose it', and 'a body at rest likes to stay at rest'. If you exercise regularly, it will benefit you in more ways than I can explain in this book about migraines. If you don't exercise regularly, you won't get those benefits. Bottom line: I highly recommend exercise.

Stress. In this day and age, we all have stress. It's not going away, and it doesn't seem to get any better. The world is short-staffed. The cost of everything is going up faster than our income. No matter your age, there are social norms and expectations causing stress in our lives. Adults are sandwiched between the needs of their children and the needs of their aging parents. The technology that is supposed to make our lives easier causes us to be on electronic devices longer and longer and we lose track of "me time".

Stress has major impacts on our bodies - both mentally and physically. Mentally it can lead to anxiety and depression. Physically it can lead to high blood pressure, gastrointestinal upset, diabetes, obesity, headaches, chronic pain conditions, stroke and heart attack, and autoimmune illness. The thing about stress is that it is usually a downward spiral. When people are stressed, it triggers migraines. The more migraines a person has, the more stress they experience…which leads to more headaches and more stress. Hence, the downward spiral. Stress can actually *create* physical symptoms. Essentially this is our brain sending a signal that we need to slow down.

Since we can't easily give up our stressful jobs or family members (like we would with foods that trigger us), we need to find constructive ways to deal with stress. Oftentimes, my patients admit to coping with stress by drinking alcohol or using tobacco, which are not healthy coping skills, and both will increase your risk of migraines, not to mention all of the other negative health effects (stroke, heart attack, cancer, etc.). The better thing is to find healthy coping mechanisms.

    Healthy ways to learn to manage stress can include physical and mental techniques. Physical techniques to reduce stress include activities like yoga, tai chi or qigong, as well as the other more active types of exercise listed previously. Mental techniques for reducing stress can include meditation, prayer, journaling, breathing exercises, and talking about your stress with another trusted human being. Talking to another person can be either sharing your stressors with a trusted friend or family member, or with a trained professional.

Psychotherapy comes in many forms - traditionally we know about meeting with therapists in person, but technology has given rise to apps where you can communicate with a therapist at your convenience. Psychotherapy is important to work through past traumas that may be still causing stress in your life, as well as helping you through current stressors from work and home life.

Chapter 3: What about genetics?

I mentioned in the introduction that migraines run strong in my family. I'm the youngest of 5 children - we all have migraines. Our mother suffered from severe migraines. And some of our children have also developed migraines. When there is a genetic component, it throws another wrench into trying to get rid of them. I've heard that some of my neurology colleagues will tell their patients that if they have a genetic cause, they are pretty much out of luck. I don't share that belief. Yes, it will cause more difficulty, but it's not impossible to gain some control over your migraines.

There is debate as to whether these are true genetic factors or if the environment plays a role, but I would argue that it's not either/or - they go together. There are several gene mutations that have been associated with migraines, meaning if you have one of these mutations you are at higher risk of experiencing migraines. Environment is also a factor because having the genetics for something doesn't mean you will express the gene. Changes in hormones and stress will change how your genes are expressed. The other part of the environmental association is what and how we eat. If we eat foods that are more likely to trigger inflammation, this will increase the likelihood of experiencing migraines, whereas if we change our diet compared to our parents, we may not have the migraines our parents did.

Genetics have always been a fascinating area of medicine for me. There are parts of our genetics that we have no control over - we can't really control the color of our eyes or how tall we are, for example. But other parts of our genetics may put us at more risk for things happening. Increased risk, however, does not equate to having the thing happen. If you make better life choices than your parents, you can prevent some of those at-risk things from happening. Stroke is an example. My mother had a stroke, which puts me at higher risk. I, however, am combating this risk by managing the risk factors that I can control such as my diet and exercise, which in turn affects my blood pressure and vascular health. We know better now, so we should do better.

Chapter 4: Let's talk about typical medication treatment

For most of my working life as a nurse and nurse practitioner, I have dealt with traditional Western medicine where we prescribe medications to treat ailments. Medical management of migraines includes various steps depending on where the patient presents. Treatment can be separated into preventive medications, acute abortive medications (abortive = stop the migraine), and emergency medication treatments (used when home therapies don't work, typically administered in the emergency room). This chapter will discuss these medications.

Preventive medications. If you are someone who struggles with frequent migraines, meaning you have many headache days per month, you may benefit from daily preventive medication. The theory behind preventive medication is that you actually prevent the migraines from happening, so you don't need to use the abortive medications or end up in the emergency room (ER). When we consider preventive medication, there are generally three classes of medications we use: antiepileptics (anti-seizure), antidepressants, and cardiac medications (typically used for blood pressure or heart rhythm management). The doses of these medications are typically smaller for migraine than they would be used for the other reasons.

There is no cookie-cutter approach to medicating a migraine patient. The provider will look at other considerations, such as whether you have any issues with depression or anxiety (might be better to start with this class of medication), if you have high blood pressure (may be best to start with a cardiac medication), or if you have low blood pressure (may be best *not* to start with a cardiac medication). If one medication doesn't work or causes too many side effects, you switch to another medication. The not-so-fun part of this is experimenting until you find something that works, which takes time and potentially lots of side effects along the way.

Since I moved away from working in the clinic, there is now another class of medications to prevent migraines - these are monthly injectable medications. If patients have tried the above oral (pill form) medications without success, these new injectable medications may be better options. I've heard really good results from many people with these, but not prescribed them or tried them myself.

Abortive medications. There are generally two classes of abortive medications: triptans and ergotamines. Triptans get their name from the ending of their generic names. These include sumatriptan, rizatriptan, etc. These medications need to be taken at the start of a migraine in order to be truly effective. If you have auras prior to the start of a migraine, this is the perfect time to use a triptan to abort (stop) the migraine from moving forward. From personal experience, if you wake up with the migraine, oftentimes these medications will not kill the migraine. You can take another dose of the medication 2 hours after the first dose if the migraine has not been fully aborted, however, you can only use these medications a max of three times in 24 hours, and insurance will only cover nine pills in a month.

    Having migraines increases your risk of suffering a stroke, as we'll talk about later in this book. One of the unfortunate outcomes of this is that once you've had a stroke, you can no longer use triptan medications to treat migraines. Triptan medications can lead to further constriction of blood vessels, leading to increased risk of stroke in patients who have already had a stroke. So, being the practitioner working with these patients in the hospital, we have lengthy conversations about what to do now that patients cannot use their favorite stroke treatment anymore.

Ergot alkaloids (ergotamine and dihydroergotamine) may be another option if patients don't tolerate triptan medications, however they can further increase risk of blood vessel constriction (narrowing), so would still not be great options for people who have had strokes.

Alternatively, if patients cannot use the triptans or ergot alkaloids or they do not work, other abortive medications include either over-the-counter Excedrine, as mentioned earlier, which is a combination of acetaminophen, aspirin, and caffeine, or a prescription medication called fioricet, which is a combination of acetaminophen, butalbital, and caffeine. Some people find relief with nonsteroidal anti-inflammatory drugs (NSAIDs) such as acetaminophen alone (Tylenol), or ibuprofen. The thing to be cautious about with using any of these medications is not to overuse them. Daily use of any of these medications can lead to rebound headaches, meaning if you try to go a day without them, you will end up with a headache because your body has gotten used to having the medication present. So, while it may seem 'safe' to use OTC medications, it does not come without risk.

Emergency medications. When the above treatments have not done their job and patients still experience severe migraines, they may present to the ER for additional treatment. Treatment in the ER typically consists of a combination of medications known as a "cocktail". There are a variety of medications that may be included in this migraine cocktail, which will vary slightly depending on provider experience and preference, or sometimes by facility protocols (guidelines recommended by the facility). These medications may include NSAIDs such as ketorolac (Toradol), triptans, magnesium, ergotamines, antiemetics (anti-nausea medications) such as ondansetron (Zofran) or prochlorperazine (Compazine), steroids, diphenhydramine (Benadryl), and/or possibly the anti-seizure medication depacon (valproic acid).

The combo is given through an intravenous (IV) line for rapid treatment. The cocktail can be repeated if not successful the first round, so some patients may need to be admitted for observation overnight. If this is the first time a person is seen in the ER with this severity of headache, they may also undergo diagnostic testing such as computed tomography (CT) scan or magnetic resonance imaging (MRI) to evaluate for additional medical issues that may be present.

Chapter 5: Now let's talk about non-typical non-medication treatment

While prescription medications can play a role in the treatment and prevention of migraines, there is also a role for non-prescription supplements. This is where I usually like to start with my patients because these generally don't come with the broad variety of side effects that the prescription medications do. This chapter will cover some of my favorite supplements, including magnesium, vitamin D, B vitamins, curcumin/turmeric, and Co-Q10.

Magnesium. While magnesium is often included in a 'migraine cocktail' given in ER and hospital settings, it is also a very useful preventive supplement. Studies do show that patients who experience migraine tend to be low in magnesium. In all honesty, magnesium levels can be hard to measure appropriately. The typical blood level of magnesium that is ordered by your primary care provider generally does not accurately reflect the available magnesium in your system. I learned years ago to measure the RBC magnesium - this measures the amount of magnesium actually in the red blood cells that are circulating in your body, or what is actually available. This level is often low, even though the 'traditional' magnesium level is "normal" - this alternate test is a much more accurate reading.

I have found that virtually all of my patients have benefited from adding magnesium to their daily routines, but especially female patients. Magnesium can be beneficial for patients that experience menstrual migraines, which we discussed earlier as hormonal-related migraines that may occur in relation to menstrual cycles.

The main side effect of magnesium is diarrhea or loose stools. This tends to be dose-specific, meaning the higher the dose, the more likelihood of experiencing bowel related side effects. There are several forms of magnesium that can be purchased OTC. The most common form is magnesium oxide. For many people, this form is just fine, but in my practice, I have found that the oxide form of magnesium tends to cause more of the unpleasant gastrointestinal (GI) effects of loose stools than other forms.

Magnesium glycinate, in my personal and professional experience, causes far less loose stools than oxide and is generally better absorbed. One of the nice things about magnesium is that it is virtually impossible to overdose on it - as you increase the dose, you have looser and looser bowel movements, so GI discomfort will generally prevent you from taking too much. For people who are prone to constipation, this supplement tends to have multiple benefits. I generally recommend starting at 400 mg daily, taken at night. That dose can be increased to about 1000 mg daily, again, dose to the stool consistency.

Vitamin D. Depending on where you live, you may or may not be more prone to vitamin D deficiency (lack of vitamin D), and this deficiency is noted to be present in 45-100% of migraine sufferers. The sun is our only natural form of vitamin D, and those that live in northern climates where it is colder and there is less daylight in the winter (thanks to the rotation of the earth) tend to be deficient just by virtue of not getting enough exposure to sunlight. Decades ago, vitamin D started being added to foods, with these foods marketed as "fortified", however the amount in these foods generally is not sufficient to maintain healthy levels of vitamin D in the body. Additionally, because milk is often the most common source of vitamin D fortified foods, there were several reports of hypercalcemia (too much calcium) in people who drank too much milk in order to try to supplement their vitamin D needs.

The vitamin D we absorb through our skin from sunlight comes in the form of vitamin D3. This form is more readily able to be used in the body than the commonly used vitamin D2, which then has to be converted into D3 for the body to use it appropriately. Additionally, vitamin D is a fat-soluble vitamin, meaning it is stored in the fat cells within our body, so it is actually possible to overdo it on this vitamin. Because of this, people may need to take a supplement daily, weekly, or even monthly, in order to maintain healthy levels of vitamin D.

Some people can take what seems like gigantic doses of vitamin D3 with little or no change in their blood levels of vitamin D. In this instance, it is recommended to take a vitamin D supplement that also includes vitamin K2. Many people know vitamin K because it is an antagonist to the blood thinner, warfarin (coumadin). Antagonist means it works against, so in this case, taking vitamin K could offset the benefit of warfarin and reverse its effects. The thing to know here is that this reversal effect is referring to K1, not K2. Vitamin K2 does not interfere with warfarin but does have a synergistic effect (working together) with vitamin D, so adding vitamin K2 to your D3 can greatly improve your absorption. Thankfully, you can purchase a supplement that includes both in one capsule, so you don't have to take two!

In general, most people need at least 2000 IU (international units, not milligrams or grams), daily. I have seen some that require up to 10,000 IU daily. This should be managed by following blood levels so you don't have too much, but to truly prevent migraines, you should be at the upper level of the recommended lab value range to really be effective. Vitamin D can provide energy, so people often take it in the morning, but it actually gives you energy by helping you sleep better, so you should take vitamin D at night so it can help stabilize your circadian rhythm.

B vitamins. There is evidence that vitamins B2, B6, and B12 can all be beneficial for migraine prevention. These vitamins are highly linked with menstrual migraines but would generally be beneficial for all types of migraines (so men can keep reading!). You can find multiple supplement options for the B vitamins OTC, but I generally do not recommend a B-complex vitamin because these typically do not have the right amount of any of the vitamins. In my personal and professional experience, I have found more benefit to supplementing just the vitamins that you are deficient in. That said, while the lab value ranges for each of these will vary slightly between labs, it is again generally best to be at the higher end of the ranges to be considered truly sufficient. Unlike vitamins D and K, the B vitamins are water-soluble, meaning you cannot truly overdo it on these, so even if you're above the range, you still won't become toxic. If you take more B vitamins than your body needs, your body will eliminate the rest through your urine (in other words, you'll have really bright yellow pee).

As far as dosing, again having blood drawn first is best, but in general vitamin B2 is recommended between 200-400 mg daily, B6 50 mg daily, and B12 at least 1000 mcg daily. These should be taken in the morning because they do help with energy right away.

Curcumin/turmeric. If you're savvy in the kitchen, you are probably familiar with the brightly yellow colored seasoning, turmeric. If you're savvy in supplements, you also know that turmeric and curcumin are nearly the same thing. Turmeric is the root of the plant that is dried and ground, whereas curcumin is extracted directly from the roots in a more complicated fashion. Both of these compounds have been proven effective for reducing inflammation, though the dried turmeric may have a slight edge on this. Turmeric has proven effectiveness in reducing specific inflammatory markers that have been connected to migraine, including calcitonine gene-related peptide (CGRP).

    Does this mean I recommend heading to your kitchen and taking in a nice big heaping spoonful of your cooking spice? The answer would be no - because it tastes terrible. I highly recommend taking it in a capsule form, with lots of water. From personal experience, if the capsule starts to dissolve in the back of your throat or upper esophagus, you will taste that flavor for far too long. Lots of water, I promise.

    Regardless of which formulation you use, curcumin or turmeric, their efficacy is boosted by another ingredient called bioperine. Bioperine comes from black pepper. By itself, it does a lot of work to prevent the body from oxidative stress from free radicals (essentially little jerks that float throughout our body causing inflammation and tissue breakdown over time). The true benefit of bioperine, however, comes from the fact that it increases the body's absorption of curcumin/turmeric. The one point of caution I would make here is that if you are one of those people that is triggered by nightshade foods, bioperine is not a supplement for you - because it also comes from the cayenne pepper family.

Co-Q10. The last (but not least) of my favorite supplements is Co-enzyme Q10, abbreviated Co-Q10. This supplement is thought to increase the energy of brain cells, and though it is unclear how exactly it works, has been shown effective at reducing migraine attacks. Dosing is recommended anywhere from 100-300 mg daily. Co-Q10 has so many benefits on the brain that I literally recommend it to virtually all of my neurological patients, regardless of the diagnosis. Honestly, that statement right there rings true for most of the supplements I just listed.

The thing you need to be cautious of with any of these supplements is where you get them and the quality of the supplements. Not all supplements are created alike. Do your research, find the best supplements for the best price that fits into your budget. The other word of advice I have with these supplements is that you don't need to add all of them, and I generally don't recommend adding them all at once - if you do that it's hard to tell which one is working. Start with one at a time, and you can always add others as you go. With the vitamins, I do generally recommend checking blood levels before starting, especially with the fat-soluble vitamin D (we don't measure K), as it is possible to get 'too much of a good thing'.

Chapter 6: What foods you *should* eat

We previously discussed things to *avoid* in your diet, now let's talk about what you *should* include in your diet. You absolutely should eat as healthy as you possibly can, meaning, eat whole, real foods as much as possible. Fresh fruits and vegetables, limited dairy (the latest statistics suggest that approximately 68% of all people are lactose intolerant), grass-fed meats whenever possible, and sustainably sourced fish. When it comes to fruits and vegetables, some of these are best purchased organic when at all possible, and some are ok to purchase non-organic. Generally, there is a list of what is called the 'dirty dozen' and 'clean 15' for which fruits should be organic and which are ok non-organic, respectively. The other consideration is whether you have diabetes or pre-diabetes. In these instances, it's best to limit your fruits to no more than 2 servings daily, because even though these are natural sugars, they are still sugars and can still wreak havoc on your body.

The old saying 'you are what you eat' is a bit outdated. I usually refer to it as 'you are what your food eats', hence the recommendation for grass-fed meats. Corn is very inflammatory to the body, and while it is not often a direct trigger for migraines, it does increase the inflammation overall in your body, which can lead to migraines. If you eat meat and your meat comes from farms where they fed the cows and chickens corn, you are getting the results of that diet. Corn is not their original source of food, so it can cause inflammation in the animal, which in turn will increase inflammation in your body. On the flip side, if they eat grass (which is their original food source), they will be healthier, and so will the meat and poultry you put into your dinner.

    I generally agree with the nutritional experts that tell us to 'eat the rainbow' because each type of food has various nutrients that we need for a healthy diet. If you limit yourself to a few staples all the time, you will be missing some of these very important nutrients. This concern comes up often when my patients tell me they are vegetarians or vegans. I understand that people will avoid meat for personal or religious reasons, but I caution people to make sure they are taking vitamins, then, to make up for the nutrients they are missing.

The other ingredient to ensure you have in your diet is protein. This, again, is a conversation that takes even more importance for those that do not eat meat or meat products, but it is true for all, as the general population typically does not get enough protein. There are a variety of protein calculators online, but they all generally ask the same questions. They want to know your age, gender, height, weight, and activity level. The results of these calculators will tell you how much protein you should take in daily given the limited information you provided. They also generally give you a list of common foods to eat to obtain the appropriate protein amounts. Foods that are high in protein include: animal products such as eggs, chicken/turkey, red meat, and fish/shellfish; nuts such as almonds and peanuts/peanut butter; dairy products including cottage cheese, Greek yogurt, milk (again see the note about dairy above); and a variety of other foods including lentils, quinoa, pumpkin seeds, and protein powders.

Over the years I started compiling a list of foods that were better than others from all of the resources I read. I no longer remember each individual resource, but I put it all in a nice little table, identifying in each food group which were better choices and which foods should be avoided. I'll include this table so you can take a look for yourself. And because this book is not very large (you'll need a magnifying glass to read the table well), I'll also include a link to the Google document so you can print yourself a larger copy if you'd like - this will be found at the end of the book.

I found, personally, that when I started by switching out some of the foods for healthier ones, it was easier than trying to make one big leap in my diet all at once. My patients also agreed that swapping out one thing for another off the list made it seem not so daunting.

Nutrition Recommendations

Food Group	Recommended	NOT Recommended	Amounts
Protein	• Grass-fed red meats when possible (beef, venison, port) - 1-2 times per week • Wild caught fish when possible (salmon, tuna) - 1-2 times per week • Free range poultry when possible (chicken, turkey)	• Deep fried meats	• Serving size about ½ cup • 3-5 servings daily depending on weight
Vegetables	• Majority of your diet, organic when possible • Leafy greens, variety • Fresh or flash-frozen • Sweet potatoes/yams	• Canned vegetables • Limit starchy vegetables (white potatoes, corn)	• Serving size about 1 cup raw • 5-7 servings daily
Fruit	• Berries (lowest in sugar)	• Fruit juices	• Serving size about 1 cup • 2 servings or less daily if diabetic • 3-4 servings for non-diabetics
Grains/ Carbohydrates	• Sprouted grain bread • Sourdough	• White break • Boxed cereals • Most granola bars	• Serving size about ¼ cup or 1 slice of bread • 2-4 servings daily
Fats	• Coconut oil • Extra virgin olive oil • Grass-fed butter (Kerrygold brand recommended) • Avocado/Avocado oil • Nut butters (except peanut butter) • Nuts (almonds, cashews)	• Vegetable oil • Canola • Margarine • Butter spreads • Peanuts/peanut butter if trying to decrease inflammation	• Serving size about 1 Tbsp • Nuts/nut butters limit to 2-3 servings daily • Include at least one at each snack/meal
Dairy	• Full fat dairy products, organic when possible	• Skim milk (high in sugar)	• If drinking milk, limit to 24 oz daily • Cheese: serving size about ¼ cup
Beverages	• Water • Red wine (4 oz) • Coffee in moderation	• Soda (diet or regular) • White whine • Fruit juices	• Water: drink about half your body weight in oz of water • Wine: max 1-2 daily • 1 cup water for every cup coffee

Mandi Counters, MSN, FNP-BC, RN, CNRN, SCRN
Nurse Practitioner/Health Coach/Podcaster
Brain Wellness Solutions
https://brainwellnesssolutions.com

Chapter 7: How about some outside-the-box treatments?

If you're a person who has tried nearly everything to reduce your migraines, you may be on the lookout for something else…there's got to be something else. This was me at one point - I thought I had exhausted all efforts and I was destined to a life of migraines because it was in my genes. I started looking for other things I could do, and the learning didn't stop. Several years ago, in my own health journey I was diagnosed with autoimmune illness and was referred to a functional medicine provider. This was a whole direction of medicine that I had never heard of. I was skeptical but open to seeing if there were other options because there *had to be something else.*

At my first functional medicine appointment, we spent over 2 hours diving into every detail of my life, from my mother's health when she was pregnant with me, all the way up to current day concerns. We talked about my sleep, my stress, any illnesses or surgeries I had in the past, and so much more. Then we ran a lot of tests to find out what kind of exposures I had had and what my genetic information could add to the diagnosis, which included providing a sample of virtually every bodily function you can capture (blood, urine, stool, saliva). Through that process, I realized there were so many avenues of health that I wasn't taught in nursing school or nurse practitioner school.

I walked away from those months of working with the functional medicine office knowing what kinds of foods would be better or worse for me based on my genetics, the knowledge that I had the genetics of someone with Celiac, clarification of vitamin and hormone deficiencies I had, and clarification that stress was a major factor for my current state of ill-health.

From there my personal search continued for other modalities of treating not only my own illnesses, but for offering other ideas to my patients. So here we are.

Some of the non-traditional treatment ideas that I have learned about and will share with you in this chapter include essential oils, daith piercing, Botox injections (this one may be more familiar for you), ozone therapy, and neurofeedback.

Essential oils. I used to think essential oils were too woo-woo - there's no way they could actually work. Well, I was wrong. I now have several bottles of lavender oil in various locations of my house. Lavender just happens to be one of the leading essential oils for headache treatment. The other oils that can be helpful for headache and pain in general include peppermint, eucalyptus, and rosemary.

There are several ways that essential oils can be used. First, essential oils can be used directly on the skin in very small amounts - I will put a drop of the oil on my finger and rub it into my temples or on my chest. You need to do this cautiously, however, as some of the oils can be harsh on the skin. If you plan to do more than a drop, or you previously noted some skin irritation with the oil directly on your skin, then the oil should be added to a carrier, such as liquid coconut oil or unscented lotion, prior to applying directly on the skin.

    Another way to use oils is to diffuse them into the air. This can be done via use of a diffuser machine - these are small and fairly portable as you can unplug them and move them from space to space. You add water and a few drops of the oil to the machine, which creates a mist in the air. You can also create a compress by means of a heated damp cloth or one of those reusable packs with rice or beads inside that can be heated and a few drops of the oil added to the compress. These can be placed on the forehead or back of neck, and not only do you get the aromatherapy from the oil, but also the heat from the compress to provide additional comfort. Lastly, you can add a few drops to a warm bath - I also like to add some Epsom salts or magnesium salts to the bath, to get even more relaxation and tension release from the bath.

Again, I give the caveat that you should do some research and make sure you are obtaining these oils from reputable sources and that they are quality oils. Not all oils are created alike, just like I mentioned with the vitamin supplements previously.

Daith piercing. A daith piercing is done in a specific fold of cartilage within your ear - not on the outer lobe of the ear as with most typical piercings. The theory behind this piercing is that acupressure can be useful for treatment of migraines, and this fold of cartilage is believed to be an acupressure point for migraine treatment. Most often people who suffer from migraines have headaches that originate on one side of their head, though sometimes they may vary from one side to the other. Generally, the daith piercing is done on the side of the head where most migraines originate. Some people who experience migraines on both sides of their head will pierce one side, and then get the other side done once the first heals and they have received benefit from the first piercing.

Because of the complexity of the acupressure point, and the difficulty of piercing this cartilage area, this piercing is at increased risk for infections and can take months to heal. It is important to research locations that do this piercing to ensure they have someone ideally who is trained and certified in this piercing technique, and that you do the proper care of your piercing to prevent frequent infections.

This is one of those alternative treatments that I looked at for quite some time before taking the plunge. I made modifications to my diet, have kept myself on all of the important supplements, yet stress is still a trigger for me, and while I try to control the things I can, I cannot control every aspect of my life, and hence I have continued to have occasional migraines. In the summer of 2022, I made an appointment at a nearby tattoo/piercing salon and walked in with a whopper of a headache. My piercing artist was quite pleased to learn that I had a migraine and promised me that I would leave without one. The skeptic in me rolled my eyes…hard. I thought there was no way he could take away my migraine that easily. Well, I was wrong again. I walked out of his salon without a headache, and my migraines have been significantly reduced since that time.

Botox injections. This alternative treatment is likely more familiar to you, and the benefit of this one is that it is often covered by health insurance now. Many years ago, it became a viable option for patients who were not experiencing relief from their migraines with all of the other pharmaceutical options given to them.

In order to qualify for Botox injections for migraine, the migraine sufferer has to try multiple medications and fail them and have enough headache days in a month to justify the treatment. This is again where that headache diary comes in handy - you need to document greater than 15 headache days per month. You also need to have documented attempting at least 2 other preventive medications from at least 2 different preventive classes. Remember those classes we talked about previously - the seizure medications, the antidepressants, and the cardiac medications. You need to have tried at least one medication from 2 different classes and have documented that they didn't work.

Once you have met these requirements, you can pursue an application with your insurance company to get Botox therapy for migraines covered. This is not your ordinary Botox injections that are used for cosmetic reasons - there is a protocol with locations specific to migraine therapy. The injections are administered every 3 months, and it is not uncommon for patients to leave the initial session without improvement in their migraines - often it takes several months to start noticing improvement.

Ozone therapy. This is the newest therapy to me, and one that I find incredibly fascinating.

Just what is ozone? Instead of the oxygen that we breathe (O2), ozone (O3) is also a gas, which is heavier than the O2 that we breathe. Ozone therapy can be administered in several ways, depending on the treatment indication. It can be injected into a muscle for pain treatment, for example. For migraine, it is injected into a patient using an IV. This requires a blood draw from the patient first. The blood taken from the patient is added together with the ozone gas and an anticoagulant (blood thinner - to prevent the blood from clotting prior to going back into the patient) and administered through an IV infusion.

When a patient first starts getting this treatment, smaller concentrations of ozone are used to determine how the patient will respond. The concentration and amounts can increase with subsequent therapies as the patient tolerates, until the maximum dose is achieved.

I have seen this administered, as well as tried it myself. If you've ever taken 'a hit' off of a helium balloon, you can relate to the slightly 'high' sensation that comes with infusion of ozone (but without the fun voice changes, darn it!). Though several research articles highlight the benefits of this therapy, it is still controversial, and you must do your research and ensure you are getting the infusions from a reputable source. The ozone used must be medical grade, so your practitioner needs to be trained in the use of the equipment.

Neurofeedback. This is another treatment I recently learned about and am incredibly fascinated with. If you are familiar with biofeedback at all (use of electrodes on muscles often alongside guided meditation - used for musculoskeletal pain treatment), then you'll find this one intriguing, as well. Neurofeedback uses quantitative electroencephalography (Q-EEG), which monitors brain wave activity, similar to if you were being evaluated for possible seizures. The patient has measurements of Q-EEG at the beginning and end of therapy, as well as sometimes periodically while undergoing treatment to evaluate the efficacy of the treatment. This is one of the easiest therapies I've ever heard of, because you literally get to sit and watch movies while your brain is being retrained to not be overly sensitive, essentially.

Other. There are so many other 'alternative therapies' for migraine prevention and treatment that this chapter could be an entire book in itself. Some of these other therapies include acupuncture, acupressure, biofeedback, massage/relaxation, CBD oil, and literally many others that you can find in a simple Google search. There are also several surgical options listed for migraine treatment - but the purpose of this book is not to highlight the surgical treatment, but identify all of the ways you can prevent the migraines from happening, and bring your attention to some of the other options you may not have thought of before for treating those sneaky little migraines that like to linger long after you've made some amazing lifestyle changes.

If you do a Google search, you'll also find the question of whether medical marijuana can be useful for migraine treatment. My long and short answer to this is yes...and no. Chronic pain is, indeed, an indicator for possible certification for medical marijuana use. On the flip side, the smell of marijuana can trigger migraines for some people. And again, the purpose of this book is to get you out of the spiral of chronic pain and help you find lifestyle management techniques to prevent the migraines, not to numb the pain away.

Chapter 8: What's the risk of not treating?

It's just a headache, right? What's the risk of having it? The list is short, but significant. One of the simplest things that can happen when you have chronic headaches and migraines is that you start taking OTC treatments daily to knock down the headache. While this may not seem like a problem (they are OTC, after all, how harmful can they be?), this can lead to rebound headaches. Meaning, if you try to go a day without your trusty OTC medication (ibuprofen, acetaminophen, etc.), your body will *create* a headache so that you will have to treat it again.

Other risks of having chronic migraines include developing a chronic pain syndrome, or hypersensitivity to pain throughout your body that is often termed fibromyalgia. Chronic pain can lead to increased blood pressure readings, which can turn into a diagnosis of hypertension (high blood pressure), which, in turn, increases your risk of many other health conditions. On a lesser scale, some people with chronic migraines will develop seizures or seizure disorder from the chronic firing of electricity in the brain.

On a scarier note, migraines increase your risk of experiencing a stroke. Research articles give a range of increased risk percentage, but in general, those who suffer chronic migraines have about twice as many strokes as people without migraines. If you have migraine with aura, this increases your risk further, as well as if you are female (our hormones tend to predispose us, apparently), and if you are on oral birth control or smoke tobacco. So, if you are a female who is on oral birth control and smokes tobacco and you have migraines with aura - you better be doing all that you can to reduce your other risks of stroke, because you need to be on high alert. That said, this is a modifiable risk factor for stroke, meaning if you take action with lifestyle management and reduce your migraines, you ultimately decrease your risk of stroke.

That's a wrap

So, now you know some of my favorite things to talk about with migraine patients. If you've been struggling with migraines forever (why else would you be reading this book?), I feel your pain, and hopefully I feel your pain reducing. I generally make no guarantees when it comes to prevention of illness, but there are actually so many things you can do to prevent migraines, that in this instance it's a pretty fair guarantee that you'll see improvement if you implement even one of the techniques discussed in this book.

I know I only said it a couple of times, but many of the things I mentioned are simple but not easy. You must have a desire to make changes. That's something I can't do for you. I can offer you the information, but you have to take it from here. If you choose to add in any of the supplements we spoke about, please let your healthcare provider know, as these still can interfere with prescription medications.

I like to explain the 'why' of anything I recommend, because I feel if you know the why, you'll be more compelled to make a change. That said, you need to know your *own* 'why'. Why do you want to get better? Why do you want less headaches? If you know this 'why', you're more likely to stick with your lifestyle changes. There will be times you don't *want* to follow more strict diets - trust me, I know this! But if you do, you'll feel better. I used to "cheat" on my diet if something was reportedly good enough (i.e., "worth it") to do so...then I started to pay for it for longer and longer periods of time. It's no longer 'worth it' to cheat on my diet.

I wish you the best in your journey. Cheers to less migraines!

MANDI
COUNTERS, NP

Nutrition Recommendations guide

Please help yourself to a copy of my Nutrition Recommendations from this link as a free gift for purchasing this book

https://docs.google.com/document/d/1M9iJFwxW3KPdTNsX58fD1CQpO6QWnUVpk3AAdT730-s/edit?usp=sharing

MANDI
COUNTERS, NP

References

Chapter 1:

1. Mayo Clinic. (2023, Feb 13). Migraine. https://www.mayoclinic.org/diseases-conditions/migraine-headache/symptoms-causes/syc-20360201

Chapter 2:

1. Caplan, L. (2009). Nonatherosclerotic vasculopathies. Caplan's Stroke (4th Ed.). Retrieved 2/14/23 from https://www.sciencedirect.com/topics/medicine-and-dentistry/vascular-headache#:~:text=Although%20migraine%20most

%20likely%20begins,part%20of%20the%20migraine%20syndrome.&text=A%20genetic%20tendency%20for%20migraine,vasoconstriction%20plays%20an%20important%20role.

2. Celiac Disease Foundation. (2023, Feb 13). What is gluten? https://celiac.org/gluten-free-living/what-is-gluten/

3. de la Monte, S. & Wands, J. (2008). Alzheimer's disease is type 3 diabetes – Evidence reviewed. *Journal of Diabetes Science and Technology.* Retrieved 2/13/23 from https://www.ncbi.nlm.nih.gov/pmc/articles/PMC2769828/

4. Diamond, M. & Marcus, D. (2016). Migraine triggers: Diet and headache control. *American Migraine Foundation.* Retrieved 2/13/23 from

https://americanmigrainefoundation.org/resource-library/diet/

5. Gundry MD Team. (2019). A comprehensive list of "deadly" nightshades. *Gundry MD*. Retrieved 2/14/23 from https://gundrymd.com/nightshade-vegetables/

6. Mayo Clinic. (2023, Feb 14). Stress management. https://www.mayoclinic.org/healthy-lifestyle/stress-management/in-depth/stress-symptoms/art-20050987#:~:text=Indeed%2C%20stress%20symptoms%20can%20affect,heart%20disease%2C%20obesity%20and%20diabetes.

7. National Sleep Foundation. (2023, Feb 13). What is REM sleep? https://www.thensf.org/what-is-rem-sleep/

8. Sleep Foundation. (2023, Feb 13). Melatonin dosage: How much melatonin should you take. https://www.sleepfoundation.org/melatonin/melatonin-dosage-how-much-should-you-take#:~:text=Doses%20of%2010%20milligrams%20or,and%20vivid%20dreams%20or%20nightmares.

9. Sleep Foundation. (2023, Feb 13). Sleep statistics. https://www.sleepfoundation.org/how-sleep-works/sleep-facts-statistics

10. Water Science School. (2019). The water in you: Water and the human body. *USGS*. Retrieved 2/14/23 from https://www.usgs.gov/special-topics/water-science-school/science/water-you-water-and-human-body#:~:text=In%20adult%20men%2C%20about%2060,their%20bodies%20made%20of%20water.

Chapter 3:

1. The Migraine Trust. (2023, Feb 16). Genetics and migraine: The role genetics play in migraine. https://migrainetrust.org/understand-migraine/genetics-and-migraine/#:~:text=Genetics%20play%20a%20big%20role,can%20bring%20on%20an%20attack.

Chapter 4:

1. Cleveland Clinic. (2023, Feb 17). When should you go to the ER for a migraine? https://health.clevelandclinic.org/should-you-ever-go-to-the-er-for-a-migraine/

2. Kurth, T. & Diener, H. (2012). Migraine and stroke: Perspectives for stroke physicians. *Stroke*. Retrieved 2/16/23 from

https://www.ahajournals.org/doi/pdf/10.1161/strokeaha.112.656603#:~:text=Migraine%20Treatment%20After%20Stroke&text=Ergotamine%20or%20triptan%20use%20is,their%20potential%20to%20narrow%20arteries.

3. Mayo Clinic. (2023, Feb 27). Headache medicine ergot-derivative-containing (Oral route, parenteral route, rectal route). https://www.mayoclinic.org/drugs-supplements/headache-medicine-ergot-derivative-containing-oral-route-parenteral-route-rectal-route/description/drg-20070161#:~:text=Dihydroergotamine%20and%20ergotamine%20belong%20to,pain%20other%20than%20throbbing%20headaches.

4. Mayo Clinic. (2023, Feb 17). Butalbital, acetaminophen, and caffeine (Oral route). https://www.mayoclinic.org/drugs-supplements/butalbital-acetaminophen-and-caffeine-oral-route/description/drg-20075393

Chapter 5:

1. American Academy of Neurology. (2004). Study shows coenzyme Q10 may prevent migraine. Retrieved 2/20/23 from https://www.aan.com/PressRoom/Home/PressRelease/185

2. American Migraine Foundation (2021). Magnesium and migraine. Retrieved 2/17/23 from https://americanmigrainefoundation.org/resource-library/magnesium/

3. Ghorbani, Z., Rafiee, P., Fotouhi, A, Haghighi, S., Magham, R., et al. (2020). The effects of vitamin D supplementation on interictal serum levels of calcitonin gene-related peptide (CGRP) in episodic migraine patients: post hoc analysis of a randomized double-blind placebo-controlled trial. The Journal of Headache and Pain. Retrieved 2/17/23 from https://thejournalofheadacheandpain.biomedcentral.com/articles/10.1186/s10194-020-01090-w#:~:text=It%20was%20estimated%20that%20about,and%20headaches%20frequency%20%5B8%5D

4. Healthline. (2023, Feb 20). Why turmeric and black pepper is a powerful combination. https://www.healthline.com/nutrition/turmeric-and-black-pepper

5. Just vitamins. (2023, Feb 20). What's the difference between turmeric and curcumin? https://www.justvitamins.co.uk/blog/whats-the-difference-between-turmeric-and-curcumin/#:~:text=So%20what's%20the%20difference%3F,known%20as%20a%20carotenoid%20compound.

6. National Headache Foundation. (2023, Feb 17). Vitamin B-2. https://headaches.org/vitamin-b-2/

7. Rezaei, S. Askari, G., Khorvash, F., Tarrahi, M. & Amani, R. (2021). Effects of curcumin supplementation on clinical features and inflammation, in migraine patients: A double-blind controlled, placebo randomized clinical trial. *International Journal of Preventive Medicine*. Retrieved 2/20/23 from

https://www.ncbi.nlm.nih.gov/pmc/articles/PMC8724631/

8. van Ballegooijen, A., Pilz, S., Tomaschitz, A., Grubler, M., & Verheyen, N. (2017). The synergistic interplay between vitamins D and K for bone and cardiovascular health: A narrative review. *International Journal of Endocrinology*. Retrieved 2/17/23 from https://www.ncbi.nlm.nih.gov/pmc/articles/PMC5613455/

9. Walk-in Lab. (2023, Feb 17). Magnesium blood test, RBC. https://www.walkinlab.com/products/view/magnesium-rbc-blood-test#:~:text=The%20RBC%20blood%20test%2C%

20also,might%20have%20a%20magnesium%20deficiency.

Chapter 6:

1. Healthline. (2023, Feb 16). 16 Delicious high protein foods. https://www.healthline.com/nutrition/high-protein-foods#The-bottom-line
2. National Institute of Diabetes and Digestive and Kidney Diseases. (2023, Feb 16). Definition & facts for lactose intolerance. https://www.niddk.nih.gov/health-information/digestive-diseases/lactose-intolerance/definition-facts

Chapter 7:

1. American Migraine Foundation (2017). Daith piercings & migraine. Retrieved 2/20/23 from https://americanmigrainefoundation.org/articles/daith-piercings-101/

2. Cleveland Clinic. (2022). Ozone therapy: What it is and why it's risky. Retrieved 2/23/23 from https://health.clevelandclinic.org/ozone-therapy/

3. Hamad, G. (2022). Ozone therapy in migraine: A potential solution. Leicester Ozone Clinic. Retrieved 2/23/23 from https://www.leicester-ozone.co.uk/post/ozone-therapy-in-migraine-a-potential-solution

4. Medical News Today. (2023, Feb 20). 5 of the most effective essential oils for headaches.

https://www.medicalnewstoday.com/articles/319478#_noHeaderPrefixedContent

5. Robinson, M. (2022). Botox for migraines: Everything you need to know. Retrieved 2/20/23 from https://www.goodrx.com/botox/botox-injections-for-migraines-side-effects-insurance-costs

6. Walker, J. (2011). Q-EEG guided neurofeedback for recurrent migraine headaches. *Clinical EEG and Neuroscience*. Retrieved 3/8/23 from https://pubmed.ncbi.nlm.nih.gov/21309444/

Chapter 8:

1. North Suffolk Neurology. (2021). Health risk of unmanaged migraines. Retrieved 2/23/23 from https://www.northsuffolkneurology.com/blog/health-

risk-of-unmanaged-migraines-27844.html#:~:text=Chronic%20Pain%3A%20Migraine%20increases%20your,migraine%20disorder%20at%20higher%20rates.

2. Oie, L., Kurth, T., Gulati, S., & Dodick, D. (2020). Migraine and risk of stroke. Journal of Neurology, Neurosurgery & Psychiatry. Retrieved 2/23/23 from https://jnnp.bmj.com/content/91/6/593

MANDI
COUNTERS, NP

About the Author

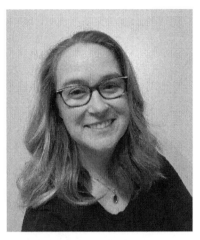

Mandi Counters is a health coach and Board-Certified Nurse Practitioner with 20+ years of experience as a Registered Nurse, 10+ of those as a Nurse Practitioner in neurosciences. Mandi has a passion for caring for patients with neurological illness, most notably stroke and migraines. Aside from being a three-time *Top Nurse Practitioner* award winner, she received the *Excellence in Teaching* award in her previous role of nursing faculty, has been on the review committee for several nursing textbooks, and holds the most prestigious award of "Best Mom Ever" from her children.

Mandi transformed her life from teen mom years ago to entrepreneur, starting Brain Wellness Solutions in 2022, a virtual neurology health coach company initially focusing on a functional medicine approach to migraine prevention and treatment, and the podcast *Brain Wellness - the Podcast*, covering all things related to brain health & wellness. Learn more at www.brainwellnesssolutions.com

Manufactured by Amazon.ca
Bolton, ON